ESSENTIAL MASSAGE OILS

THE ULTIMATE GUIDE ON THE USE OF OILS

JAMIE J.

CONTENTS

Introduction   v

1. Usage and Application Guide   1
2. How tos on Essential Oils: 4
3. Applications of Essential Oils   6
4. Other Uses   12
5. Some Highly Useful Essential Oils   14
   Afterword   23
   Sneak Peek - Chapter 1   26

©Copyright 2022 – **All rights reserved by Jamie J.**

The content of this book may not be reproduced, duplicated, or transmitted without direct written permission from the author or publisher.

ISBN-978-1-63970-127-8

Legal Notice:

This book is copyright protected. This is only for personal use. You cannot amend, distribute, sell, use, quote, or paraphrase any part of the content within this book without the consent of the author or publisher.

Disclaimer notice:

Please note the information contained within this document is for educational and entertainment purposes only.

Every attempt has been made to provide accurate, up-to-date, and reliable complete information.

No warranties of any kind are expressed or implied. Readers acknowledge that the author is not engaging in the rendering of legal, financial, medical or professional advice. The content of this book has been derived from various sources. Please consult a licensed professional before attempting any techniques outlined in this book.

By reading this document, the reader agrees that under no circumstances is the author responsible for any losses, direct or indirect, which are incurred as a result of the use of the information contained within this document, including, but not limited to, -errors, omissions, or inaccuracies.

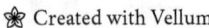 Created with Vellum

INTRODUCTION

Essential Oils are derivatives from natural sources, and these are entirely plant-related i.e. taken from kernels, rinds, flowers, seeds, and even plant parts like the bark and roots. They have therapeutic and relaxing effects when applied to the skin or just inhaled. As they are plant derivatives, Essential Oils play a vital role in perfumery and even in food processing as aromatic enhancers.

Almost all Essential Oils are highly volatile. They evaporate fast and should be stored under airtight conditions. There are many ways in which Essential Oils are extracted. Fragrance Extraction and Distillation and Steam Distillation processes have been in use from the old days itself. The newer methods, including Cold Pressing, do not use heat in the extraction process and allow maximum preservation of all the beneficial compounds seen in Essential Oils. It has become a common trend to buy Cold Pressed Oils as they offer more therapeutic value to the blends and oils used in massages.

Essential Oils are sometimes confused with Aromatic Oils. Even though both have many similar properties, Essential Oils are a complex mixture of various aromatic compounds. All Essential Oils, as they are extracted, come in highly concentrated forms, a drop of which sometimes equalling multiple grams of the herb itself. For example, a drop of Peppermint oil has the same benefits as over 25 cups of Peppermint Herbal Tea. Care should be taken when using Essential Oils, and often a prescription from an experienced practitioner is advised. People with allergies to certain types of plant products should restrain from oils derived from those ingredients.

Essential Oils are well known for their manifold health benefits as they are antibiotic, antifungal, anti-inflammatory, and even antiviral. In addition, they have curative properties on muscles, joints, and the skin, go well beyond physical benefits, have relaxing and rejuvenating impacts on the brain, and elevates one emotionally and even spiritually. Furthermore, essential oils can be blended with other Base Oils, thus volumizing them in quantity and quality.

1

USAGE AND APPLICATION GUIDE

Essential Oils are potent owing to their concentrated nature. And understanding the application and usage is quite important. This does not mean that you must take overwhelming classes to be able to use them. Just follow these essential tips that have been specially compiled for you. A thing to note here is that Essential Oils have different properties and should not use all oils the same way or for various purposes. These tips are aimed at the novice and the regular user to keep a handy note to refer. And see how to use these oils for your wellbeing and the people around you.

Personal Judgment: When it comes to tools to better understand Essential Oils, the best one and the foremost one is your nose. Your mind and intuitions play a vital role in what you use for your body, and this can take you long in the ever-widening route of knowledge. Once you know what is good for you, experiment with other oils.

Start Small: An excess of anything is harmful. The oils that we use are very potent and may be detrimental if not used wisely. If you feel confused about using new oil, read the precautions, consult a doctor, apply a small amount as a patch test and finally use the oil after diluting it to a good extend.

Reading the Label: Usually, Essential Oils come with a colored code in the label:

Green: Is generally safe for use and can be used undiluted

Orange: Safe for general use and can be used diluted moderately.

Red: Heavy dilution is required and also to consult a doctor before use.

Though the green and orange are safe, wise discretion and a doctor's advice are always better.

All Oils are Different:

Oils like Peppermint and Lemon have diverse uses in the application. But some are Topical Oils like Eucalyptus and cannot take this internally.

While it is always wise to follow precautions, a general rule is that only well-known brands publish precautions based on actual research. Brands that are cheap and not well known may not produce precautions based on research, and they also may have a lot of contaminants in them. Therefore, when using oil internally, it should take great care, and it always is better to do so under a prescription from a reputed practitioner.

HOW TOS ON ESSENTIAL OILS:

Aromatic Uses of Essential Oils:

The most common and widely used application of Essential Oils is Aromatic. They smell delicious, and so the widespread use of it aromatically. They also stimulate the Limbic System, which is responsible for the moods that often come and go. Some oils also rid us of nasal congestions.

Aromatic properties can:

Improve indoor air purity, prevent many airborne diseases, and even detoxify some of the contaminants.

Improve mood, balance hormones, and provide for emotional and spiritual well-being.

. . .

Be a complete cure for the sinuses and respiratory system.

Improve the immune system and benefit overall health.

Essential Oils are volatile, and when massaging onto the body, the fumes arising from them get to you internally through your respiratory system.

The fumes contain thousands of beneficial compounds present in the parent oil and can infuse the effects deeply into your system. The nasal sensations directly affect the Limbic system and can enhance or relax your mood.

3

APPLICATIONS OF ESSENTIAL OILS
AROMATIC APPLICATIONS

1. Diffusing: This is used to improve the air purity of your home. Essential oils can be spread or diffused in the air through many methods, and some even use Ultrasonic vibrations to do so. The aim is to spread the compounds of the oils in the air and have them over there for a longer duration. And it is so detoxifying the air and purifying it. It should be done at a moderate room temperature, and the diffuser should not be warm either; heat can diminish and even nullify the benefits of the compounds.

2. Inhalation: Done directly from the bottle itself. The fumes are inhaled through the nostrils; this is more direct and can be used, especially with congestion. It is to be noted that the bottle is placed a few inches; five is normal from your nose. These oils can be spicy at times and can irritate your nostril or even burn them a bit. The safest way is cupping, in which you add a drop of oil in your palms and cup them closely over your respiratory tracts. Frequent opening and closing of the oils is not advised as it speeds up the evaporation and the effects of the oil. Not all oils can be inhaled directly.

. . .

3. Propped Inhalation: This is often used for babies as this method does not need direct contact. A drop of Essential oil is placed in a cotton swab pillow or even the collar of the shirt and inhaled over longer duration or while sleeping. Sometimes this is also used to get a deep and proper sleep.

4. Vapour Inhalation: By far the most common method but done wrongly! Heat some water in a pot and refrain from boiling it; heat leaves the fumes less medicated to that extent. Next, cover your head with a long blanket and inhale the fumes through your nose and mouth. It is best to do this daily as it has many benefits and is especially good if you have congestion or trouble with your phlegm.

5. Humidifier: As mentioned throughout the text, heat and Essential Oils do not go well, so a humidifier with cool air is preferred. Care should be given when using a humidifier as the compounds in oils can damage parts of the humidifier. Some brands are specifically made Essential Oil Safe.

6. Vent: Essential Oils like Ginger and Peppermint can be applied on a cloth or cotton pad and placed in the vent of vehicles to prevent travel sickness.

7. Perfumery: This is a better and healthier option than chemical-based sprays and deodorants. Apply on the wrists, and behind the ears, this catches the attention of all and lingers longer than ordinary perfumes. Also, can be dissolved in water or alcohol and be applied as mist on your body.

. . .

8. Room Purifier: Rooms can get congested or smell bad sometimes. Instead of using chemicals to do odorizes, you can create one by blending half-cup alcohol and 30 drops of Essential oil in a decorative decanter. Bamboo skewers dipped in the bottle will spread the fumes lightly in the air and keep it from evaporating fast.

TOPICAL APPLICATIONS:

- Topical application is using the oil directly on the skin. Though a natural derivative, the high concentration of these oils can irritate your body. Knowing the skin type and your allergies should be kept in mind before venturing out into topical applications.

- Patch test: Apply a slight drop of diluted oil in the soft part of your arm and see if it causes redness to the skin or a bit of a tinge. If so, then you need some other oil that goes well with your skin.

- General Precautions:

1. Oils that increase skin sensitivity when exposed to sunlight should be avoided during the daytime. This is best used after sundown or onto clothed parts of the body. For example, citrus oils can increase sensitivity up to 12 hours, while bergamot can go up to 3 days.

. . .

2. There are Neat Oils that come in bottles with 'Can use Un Diluted' labels. It is best t use these oils with higher dilution first and then zeroing on the dilution rate to be completely safe from rashes.

3. If you have a routine of applying oil to your body, try blending or diluting the oil. Excessive use of the same oil may make your skin prone to rashes or allergic reactions. Also, bending helps in better absorption of the compounds of the Essential Oil.

4. Layer your oils. This is done by applying an Essential Oil first and applying another one after a gap of five minutes. Blending Oils need a good amount of technical knowhow and are not advised to the novice, but if you still want to try out a blend, always go for layering.

Common Topical Applications:

1. Massage: This is the best and most common way of using Essential Oils to the body. Oil applied to muscles and joints have a therapeutic as well as relaxing effect. Move towards the torso when massaging the arms and legs and not the other way around. Avoid firm pressure and avoid areas like the spine.

2. Spot Application: This is usually done when focusing on a specific area of the body.

3. Reflex Points: There are many reflex points in the feet and palm that correspond to various internal organs. Applying oils

here can be very beneficial as the feet and palms have tougher skin that can withstand many reactions. In addition, the lubricant applied here is infused into the bloodstream in a much better way. Professionals usually do this, but simple know-how can be of help.

4. Auricular: There are more minor pressure points around and on the ears. Massaging Lavender can relax even a child having a mood upset.

5. Compresses: If you have a joint ache or sprain, you can soak a soft cloth in warm or cold water with a few drops of specific Essential Oil, apply it on the spot, and compress it softly with your hand. This is soothing, and the oil also goes in deep to cure the damage.

6. Baths: Essential Oils can be added directly to the bath and foot baths. For itchy feet, Melaleuca is advised. It is also good to use a carrier oil to disperse the concentration of the concentrated oil all over the body than just on one part of the body.

INTERNAL APPLICATIONS:

There is no common consensus over the use of Essential Oils internally. Some say it is good, while others object to it fiercely. The truth lies amid this significant divide. It is to be remembered that Essential Oils are concentrated and to take them internally needs a lot of care and discretion. To get some negative results, you may need to ingest a large quantity, which doesn't mean that you will be critically ill. Some Essential Oils smell tasty, and like food, so it is advised to keep them out of reach from minors.

General Precautions:

1. Start with one oil, then a blend. Giving a gap of 20 minutes is always good before ingesting the oil.

2. Some Essential Oils work topically for ailments like indigestion. Internal applications should be administered as a last resort.

3. General oil consumption is limited to 10-20 drops, so if you have a routine of taking Essential Oils internally, then modify it to 15 drops is much better at ten drops.

4. Oils with high levels of Phenol (Thyme, Oregano, etc.) get stored in the liver and are not to be consumed without a prescription.

5. Always use Base Oil like coconut or olive oil to dilute Essential Oils before taking it orally.

4

OTHER USES

Cooking:
Essential Oils are regularly used in roasts and bakes. As these oils are concentrated, you need less than a drop in the preparation. Although some recipes suggest a little more than that or suggest 'according to taste', it is better to go with less than a drop at first and slowly increase it when you try it out the next time. Phenol-rich oils like Oregano are best internally when adding to the food you cook, as the heat will nullify almost all of the harmful effects.

Drinking: Adding flavors like Peppermint and citrus flavors to drinking water makes them flavorful and even energy giving and a lot of people also add them to their daily dose of milk. These are oils, and they don't generally mix well with water or milk. Give it a thorough shake before drinking it as the oil stays at the top, and the concentrated oils may burn your lips and mouth.

Supplement: Having a moderate daily dose of Essential Oils can help you digest better, feel fresh, and as a healthy chew for children. Adding less than a drop to 5 ml of honey is the best way to have it.

Around the Home Application:

Using Essential Oils for Household application is by far the safest to use. Some of the Oils are anti-bacterial and anti-fungal and are a panacea for having a spic and span household.

Using a Citrus Essential Oil while doing dishes cuts through all the grime and leaves a good after scent to the dishes.

This is also good when hanging out clothes for drying. Citrus-based oils should not be used as they increase sensitivity to light and may fade the clothes.

Citrus-based oils are also good cleansers, are very effective on gum, and are suitable for most surfaces.

Most Oil can be mixed with cleansers and used even as a dry carpet duster before vacuuming.

Some oils like Peppermint are very effective against pests and can be applied to cotton swabs and placed on parts of the house where there are chances of vermin attack.

5

SOME HIGHLY USEFUL ESSENTIAL OILS

Some Essential Oils can be stored for use for almost any purpose.

Eucalyptus Oil:

It helps dilate the circulatory system and helps in rejuvenating the entire body.

It relieves Asthmatic attacks if inhaled directly or just massaged over the chest.

It is very effective in increasing blood flow to the brain.

The topical and aromatic application directly or indirectly is good to rid bronchitis.

. . .

Rid of nasal congestion. If massaged on the chest and other areas, it relieves the effects of the common cold.

If applied in the bathtub or bathing water, it cools down the body and adds zest to your mind and muscles.

Applied by massaging on the chest and related areas, it is good medicine for coughs.

As it increases blood circulation, it is very effective against diabetes. Massaging the oil regularly on the body is very effective for people suffering from this disease.

If applied after diluting, it is good for cuts and burns as it has disinfectant properties.

Application of this oil in an anti-clockwise direction is a good remedy for dysentery.

Massaging the oil around the ear in a diluted solution is good against ear inflammation.

Emphysema is a respiratory disease that gets treated if massaged with this on the chest and related areas.

Massaged onto the chest helps melt down mucus and is a good expectorant.

. . .

It is cooling to the body, and when used on a patient having a high fever, it helps reduce the temperature and eases down congestion.

Massaging onto the soles can regulate blood sugar levels.

It stimulates the lymph glands and is good to fight inflammation.

Massaging around the temples is suitable for the irises.

Topical use or wetting a towel with this oil helps in fighting jet lag.

Massaging near the Kidney topically helps in curing Kidney stones.

Is a good medicine against lice.

Diffusing the oil in the room of the afflicted helps in curing measles.

Reduces pain resulting from Neuralgia.

Massaging with this oil reduces inflammation caused by Neuritis.

. . .

Reduces muscle fatigue and reduces the building up of lactic acid.

Reduces all kinds of pain.

Massaging and inhaling the fumes of this oil fight against pneumonia.

Diffusing this oil in the room fights against all respiratory viruses.

Fights against Rhinitis and Sinusitis.

Adding to a warm bath helps against Shingles.

If massaged by a practitioner, this is a good treatment for Tennis Elbow.

Reduces inflammation of the lungs and kills bacteria and is a good cure for tuberculosis.

It is also good to fight hay fever, acne and many types of infection.

Cilantro Oil:

. . .

Diffusing this oil in the room or using a diffuser pendant fight against ADD/ADHD. This can be applied to the sloes directly.

Inhalation of the fumes helps against fighting anxiety.

Cilantro is a good flavoring for savories and salads. Use this diluted and increase the concentration slowly.

Rubbing it in the palm ad inhaling it deeply for 20 seconds helps relieve depression. Topical and internal use can help in the detoxification of the body.

Massaging on the abdomen in a clockwise direction can help indigestion.

Added to food, it can be a supplement that enhanced flavor and strengthens the immune system.

It fights against all infections.

The oil has anti-inflammatory effects and is the first aid in sprains and related ailments.

Applied onto pillows, it helps in deeper sleep patterns.

. . .

It is used in treatments for lead poisoning.

It helps muscles to renew after soreness and overstrain.

Wild Orange Oil:

Rubbing this oil on the palms and cupping it can reduce stress and anxiety.

Rubbed on the lower abdomen and the solar plexus can add confidence.

Two drops mixed with the same amount of Base oil can relieve constipation.

Adds a fresh flavor to foods and smoothies.

Massaging on the abdomen anti-clockwise can cure all stomach upsets.

Taken internally with water or massaged onto the belly can stimulate an upset digestive system.

Rubbed near the heart can control heart palpitations.

. . .

It helps in boosting the immune system

Though this is invigorating oil, some people use it to get better sleep as it also has calming effects.

Diluted with carrier oil, it can be used to cure jaundice, especially for babies.

Massaging this around the neck helps in balanced hormone levels.

It fights against scurvy due to the high levels of vitamin C
   Cupping or diffusing through other means adds zest to your mood and energy levels.

It is also effective for muscle fatigue, tissue repair, and weight loss, and skin blemishes.

Patchouli Oil:

Patchouli Oil is a very effective deodorant and has been in use in perfumery for decades. Other than cosmetic use it has the following benefits too:

If you add this oil to your routine skin pack or rub it on the areas of concern, it will fight all the problems associated with acne.

. . .

Regular application on the soles, chest, and the back of the neck will strengthen your immune system and fight against allergies.

Cupping it over the mouth and nose helps you keep calm and reduce anxiety.

It helps soothing cancer if applied to the area.

Daily hair care application has proven anti-dandruff benefits.

It applies with a carrier oil that has moisturizing effects; this is a good cure for dermatitis.

It can be supplemented with other oils to detoxify the body.

Stimulates the urinary system as it is a good diuretic.

Help reduce fever if massaged slowly on the forehead and neck.

Soothes headache if rubbed on the temples.

It is a good remedy for wounds, snake bites, and insect bites
    A good enough repellent against termites and ants.

It can be used for all types of infections on the skin.

. . .

Rubbing it onto the back of the neck has soothing effects.

If you have stretch marks, make it a routine to apply this oil to those areas.

It has been in use for tissue regeneration by applying it diluted to areas that need repair.

It takes care of wrinkles and other problems associated with old age.

AFTERWORD

The list is endless, and it will take volumes and volumes to describe all the benefits of the infinite list of Essential Oils and their uses. Now that you know the basics of selecting and using Essential Oils, it's time to experiment! Never go ahead and apply it to your skin, especially the face, or ingest it. Al Essential Oils are concentrated, and even if you see safe to use undiluted recommendations, it's better to be wise than sorry. You may have susceptible skin, and the oil may leave rashes on your body. Always use oils diluted and slowly increase the concentration.

It's always better to consult a doctor and know what stuff you are allergic to. Then, refrain from oils or blends that use these ingredients. Always do a patch test before directly applying it to your body. Most Oils work well even if applied topically, and ingesting oils should only be done under supervision and only done as a last resort.

Essential Oils have many benefits, and many of them can be applied as a routine to your body. It also has a lot of cleansing effects on the body and around the home. These can be substituted for chemical deodorants, and the aroma they leave behind is just heavenly and can't be manipulated by chemicals.

Some of these oils can be a must-have in your home medicine kit as they are safe and have antifungal and antiseptic effects. Specially made diffusers also can come in handy if anyone has a fever or an upsetting mood.

To top it all, Essential Oils are safe and suitable. It will take multiple bottles to make you ill if you ingest it. It is a natural derivative and will never harm you and make you critical. It's always best to keep them out of reach from minors and ALWAYS use them diluted. If some oils are to be used internally, try using them as a flavoring in your food. Make Essential Oils a part of your daily life for the well-being of you and your family.

The End.

Did you like this book? Then you'll LOVE Perfect Massage Therapy: The Best Massage Tips You Wish You Knew

Learn The Best of the Best Massage Tips and Techniques!

Massages are a miraculous way to cure almost all ailments be it physical or emotional. Getting a massage and giving one can be a very intimate affair. Being the most natural way to tend to wounds and blemishes, massages have come a long way with traditions and science adding a twist here and there. Massages are getting pricier by the day and terms often confuse the layperson. This book sheds some light on all the common types of massage and over 30 tips.

Take action and grab your copy of this Massage book and learn how to relax and make your loved ones feel extremely good by learning sensual massage and massage therapy which will help you relieve pain and feel more focused.

This book here is the most complete and comprehensive guide on Massage Therapy

Click here to start reading Perfect Massage NOW!

Perfect Massage Therapy: The Best Massage Tips You Wish You Knew

https://books2read.com/u/b6Mlop

SNEAK PEEK - CHAPTER 1

Click here to start reading Perfect Massage NOW!

Perfect Massage Therapy: The Best Massage Tips You Wish You Knew

https://books2read.com/u/b6Mlop

The Erogenous Zones

The term is taken from the Greek Eros, meaning love, and Genes meaning born. Therefore, the term applies to any part of the body that has a level of sensitivity at a heightened level as there are several nerve endings. The stimulation of these parts directly or indirectly produces sexual arousal, fantasies, and even orgasm.

Erogenous zones are spread all over the body. Some areas are more sensitive than others. Depending on the body, stimulation of these parts can produce different arousal levels. To give a sensual massage, a thorough understanding of the erogenous zones is essential as an immediate orgasm may often reduce the effects of the massage.

The Erogenous zones are divided into two categories:

1. Nonspecific Zones: These areas resemble normal skin and have a lot of nerve endings that help in heightened stimulation. The nape of the neck, inner arms, etc. are some examples.
2. Specific Zones: These areas are denser in nerve endings and often cause sexual arousal. It is said that they have a close connection with the brain and the brain's reward system.

For males, the focus falls on the pubic region mainly. The erogenous zones are the areas like the top part of the glans and the sides, the side of the penis, the scrotum, the perineum, the anus, and the surrounding areas.

There are many more erogenous zones when it comes to women. The genital area of women is called the vulva. The clitoris and the outer parts of the vagina have a lot of nerve endings and can be stimulated even to reach an orgasm without penetration.

Other erogenous areas include:

1. The Scalp: A massage to the scalp or a hair caress is relaxing and yet very stimulating to many.
2. The nape of the neck is a very sensitive part and is usually aroused by kissing, biting (softly), or licking. It is an extremely sensitive zone in females and where 'love bites' are found.
3. The Ear: The outer sides of the ear and the lobe are sensitive areas that respond to licking or nibbling.
4. The Chest: The entire breast area of both men and women has several nerve endings and can be aroused using the hands. The areola and the nipples are also highly sensitive. Stimulating the hair around the areola produces oxytocin and stimulates the genital region.
5. The Abdomen: The lower part of the abdomen and the entire navel is very responsive to touch. They also stimulate the genital areas primarily due to their proximity.
6. The Arms: The softer inner parts of the arm and your elbow are extremely erogenous to both men and women.
7. The Armpits: This is a highly erogenous area, especially if it has hair on it. Slowly caressing the armpit is a very stimulating experience, and it is also believed to produce pheromones in men and women.
8. The Fingers: The fingers, especially the tips and the top cone, have an abundance of nerve endings and can be stimulated orally.
9. The Legs: The inner part of the thighs leading to the pubic region is very responsive to caresses and light massages.
10. The Feet: Especially the toes as there are a lot of nerve endings, responds to caresses and oral stimulation. The rough areas at the knees and ankles are also found to create an erogenous sensation if stimulated with soft caresses.

SENSUAL MASSAGE IN SEX THERAPY

Sensual Massage plays an important role in Sex Therapy these days. This has manifold effects on the sexual well-being of the person, but it is mainly used to stimulate and enhance their libido (positive response to sexual stimuli. It is also done by professionals on men who have premature ejaculation issues.

The use of Sensual Genital Massage refers to physicians' use to treat women having Female Hysteria. This was popular as a treatment until finally, the patients were referred to midwives. However, it was time-consuming, and the patients needed treatment regularly.

Some techniques have been derived from research that enhances orgasm in both men and women. One such technique is called Extended Orgasm. It does not come under normal orgasms but can be explained as more intense sensations that last anywhere from some minutes to an hour or more. In addition, the orgasms have been.

Neo Tantra

This is the Western modification of Tantric Sex. Tantric Sex is all about elevating sexual satisfaction to a spiritual level, whereas the former is not that much into spiritual attainment. After thorough research on the Buddhist and Hindu Tantra, the Western Neo-Tantra has come to be.

It involves all the rituals of the traditional one and has brought forth many unorthodox movements. There is also a famous school of thought called Sex Magic.

End of Sneak Peek

Click here to start reading Perfect Massage NOW!

Perfect Massage Therapy: The Best Massage Tips You Wish You Knew

https://books2read.com/u/b6Mlop

www.ingramcontent.com/pod-product-compliance
Lightning Source LLC
LaVergne TN
LVHW021743060526
838200LV00052B/3450